THE ART AND SCIENCE OF GASTRIC ULCER

ACIDIC ALCHEMY

By

Dr. Elvira S. Graves

Table of contents

Disclaimer

Introduction

Gastric ulcers, a type of peptic ulcer disease, have long been shrouded in myths and misconceptions. Commonly misunderstood as a mere consequence of stress or spicy food, the reality of gastric ulcers is far more complex and rooted in the intricate balance of the body's internal chemistry and external influences.

At its core, a gastric ulcer is a lesion in the stomach lining, a breach in the mucosal integrity due to an imbalance between aggressive factors like stomach acid and pepsin, and the defense mechanisms that protect the stomach's inner layer. This condition is not merely an inconvenience but a serious health concern that can significantly impact an individual's quality of life.

Defining Gastric Ulcers

Traditionally, gastric ulcers have been defined by their symptoms—pain, discomfort, and indigestion. However, modern medicine allows us to understand them as the result of various factors, including infection with the bacterium *'Helicobacter pylori'* (H. pylori), prolonged use of nonsteroidal anti-inflammatory drugs (NSAIDs), and other physiological and genetic factors.

Dispelling Misconceptions

One of the most enduring myths is that ulcers are caused solely by stress or eating habits. While these can exacerbate the condition, they are not the primary causes. Another common fallacy is that milk can soothe ulcers, when in fact, it may increase acid production and worsen the condition.

The True Nature of Gastric Ulcers
Gastric ulcers are a manifestation of a disease process where the delicate balance of the stomach's environment is disrupted. They are a signal that our body's natural defenses are overwhelmed, necessitating medical attention and often lifestyle changes.

In this book, **"The Art and Science of Gastric Ulcer: Acidic Alchemy,"** we will explore the multifaceted nature of gastric ulcers, from their scientific underpinnings to the art of managing and treating them. We will unravel the complexities of the gastric environment, delve into the latest research, and address the holistic approaches to healing. Join us on this journey to demystify gastric ulcers and discover the alchemy of acidity that governs our digestive well-being.

Chapter 1: Introduction to Gastric Ulcers

Understanding the Basics

Gastric ulcers, also known as stomach ulcers, are open sores that develop on the lining of the stomach. Unlike abrasions that occur on the skin, these ulcers form in an environment constantly exposed to acidic gastric juices, making them a significant medical concern. The development of a gastric ulcer is a complex process, often involving an imbalance between the stomach's aggressive digestive fluids and the defense mechanisms of its mucosal lining.

Historical Perspective

The history of gastric ulcers is a testament to the evolution of medical understanding. For centuries, ulcers were attributed to stress and poor lifestyle choices. It wasn't until the late 20th century that two Australian scientists, Barry Marshall and Robin Warren, discovered the role of Helicobacter pylori bacteria in ulcer formation, revolutionizing treatment approaches and earning them the Nobel Prize in Physiology or Medicine in 2005.

Prevalence and Demographics

Gastric ulcers affect a significant portion of the population worldwide, with variations in prevalence across different regions and demographics. Factors such as age, dietary habits, use of certain medications, and socioeconomic status play a role in the distribution of this condition. In many cases, ulcers are a manageable condition, but they can lead to serious complications if left untreated.

This chapter sets the stage for a deeper dive into the art and science of gastric ulcers, providing readers with a foundational understanding of their nature, history, and impact on human health. As we progress through the book, we will explore the complexities of diagnosis, treatment, and management, all while debunking myths and shedding light on the true 'acidic alchemy' at work in our stomachs.

The Gastric Ulcer Spectrum
Gastric ulcers are not a monolithic condition; they exist on a spectrum, ranging from mild, asymptomatic cases to severe, life-threatening emergencies. The severity of an ulcer is influenced by its location within the stomach, its size, and the presence of underlying health conditions.

The Role of Gastric Acid

Central to the development of gastric ulcers is gastric acid, a corrosive fluid composed primarily of hydrochloric acid (HCl). In a healthy stomach, this acid plays a crucial role in digestion and defense against pathogens. However, when the protective mucosal barrier is compromised, acid can attack the stomach lining, leading to ulceration.

The Impact of H. pylori

Helicobacter pylori infection is a major contributor to gastric ulcers. This bacterium can disrupt the mucosal barrier and incite inflammation, setting the stage for ulcer development. It is a common infection, yet not everyone with H. pylori will develop an ulcer, highlighting the complexity of the disease.

Lifestyle Factors

Lifestyle choices, such as smoking and alcohol consumption, can exacerbate the risk of developing gastric ulcers. These factors can impair the mucosal defenses and increase acid production, creating a hostile environment for the stomach lining.

Medications and Ulcers

Certain medications, particularly NSAIDs, can significantly increase the risk of gastric ulcers. These drugs interfere with the production of prostaglandins, substances that help maintain the protective lining of the stomach.Gastric ulcers, which are a specific type of peptic ulcer, can be classified into four main types based on their location in the stomach:

Type 1: These ulcers are located near the lesser curvature, the right border of the stomach, and are the most common type of gastric ulcer.

Type 2: Found near the duodenum or pyloric channel, Type 2 ulcers often co-occur with duodenal ulcers.

Type 3: These are located in the prepyloric region, just above the pylorus, which is the opening to the small intestine.

Type 4: Type 4 ulcers form higher up on the lesser curvature, near the cardia, which is the part of the stomach closest to the esophagus.

The symptoms of gastric ulcers can vary depending on the type. While the main symptom is typically a gnawing or burning pain in the middle of the stomach, not all ulcers are painful. Some may not cause any symptoms until they lead to complications. Types 2 and 3 ulcers can also cause excess stomach acid secretion, leading to symptoms like heartburn, acid reflux, and nausea.

It's important to note that duodenal ulcers, which form in the first part of the small intestine, are also peptic ulcers but are not classified as gastric ulcers.

The symptoms of gastric ulcers can vary from person to person, but common signs include:

 Burning stomach pain: This pain can fluctuate, often worsening with an empty stomach and improving after eating or taking antacids.

Feeling of fullness, bloating, or belching: Discomfort can occur, especially after eating.

 Intolerance to fatty foods: Fatty foods may increase discomfort and pain.

Heartburn and nausea: These are also common symptoms associated with gastric ulcers.

Vomiting or vomiting blood: This can appear red or black and is a sign of a more serious complication.

Dark blood in stools, or stools that are black or tarry: Indicative of bleeding in the stomach.

Trouble breathing: If the ulcer is causing significant pain or bleeding, it may lead to difficulty breathing.

Feeling faint: This can occur, particularly if there is significant blood loss.

Unexplained weight loss and changes in appetite: These symptoms can occur due to pain or discomfort associated with eating.

If you or someone else is experiencing severe symptoms or complications from a gastric ulcer, such as persistent vomiting, vomiting blood, or black stools, it's important to seek medical attention immediately. These could be signs of a serious condition that requires prompt treatment.

The risk factors for developing a gastric ulcer include:

Infection with *Helicobacter pylori*: This bacterium commonly lives in the mucous layer of the stomach and can cause inflammation and ulcers.

Long-term use of NSAIDs: Nonsteroidal anti-inflammatory drugs like ibuprofen and naproxen can decrease the stomach's mucous layer that protects against acid[1].

Smoking: Cigarette smoking can impair the protective lining of the stomach and increase acid production.

Alcohol consumption: Regular alcohol use can damage the stomach lining.

Stress: While not a direct cause, stress can exacerbate existing ulcers and impede healing[2].

Spicy foods: They do not cause ulcers but can aggravate symptoms[1].

Other factors: These include age, dietary habits, genetic predisposition, and the presence of other medical conditions. It's important to manage these risk factors to prevent the development of gastric ulcers or to prevent existing ulcers from worsening. If you suspect you have a gastric ulcer, it's crucial to consult a healthcare provider for proper diagnosis and treatment.

This chapter has laid the groundwork for understanding gastric ulcers, their causes, and the factors that influence their development. As we move forward, we will delve deeper into the diagnostic journey, treatment modalities, and the ongoing quest for a cure. The subsequent chapters will build upon this foundation, offering a holistic view of gastric ulcers and their management in the modern world.

Chapter 2: The Gastric Environment and Its Relation to Other Internal Organs

Anatomy of the Stomach

The stomach is a muscular, J-shaped organ that serves as a reservoir for food, initiating the digestive process. It's divided into four main regions: the cardia, fundus, body, and pylorus. Each region has specific cells that contribute to the stomach's functions, such as secreting gastric juices, hormones, and protective mucus.
The Cardia is where food enters from the esophagus. The Fundus and the Body are the main sites for mixing food with gastric secretions. The Pylorus acts as a gatekeeper,

controlling the passage of digested food into the small intestine.

Role of Acid and Pepsin
Gastric acid, primarily hydrochloric acid (HCl), creates an acidic environment with a pH of 1.5 to 3.5, which is essential for pepsin activation. Pepsin is an enzyme that breaks down proteins into smaller peptides. The secretion of gastric acid and pepsin is regulated by neural and hormonal signals in response to food intake.

Protective Mechanisms of the Gastric Mucosa
The gastric mucosa is lined with a thick layer of mucus that protects the stomach lining from the corrosive effects of acid. Bicarbonate ions secreted by epithelial cells also help neutralize the acid. Additionally, the mucosa has a rich blood supply that aids in nutrient absorption and provides cells with oxygen and energy for repair and regeneration.

Relation with Other Internal Organs
The stomach interacts with other organs to ensure efficient digestion. The liver produces bile, stored in the gallbladder and released into the duodenum to emulsify fats. The pancreas secretes digestive enzymes into the small intestine to further break down food particles. The stomach's motility is coordinated with the small intestine to regulate the rate of gastric emptying.

Certainly! Let's delve deeper into the gastric environment and its relationship with other internal organs.

Microenvironment of the Gastric Mucosa
The gastric mucosa is not just a passive barrier; it's a dynamic microenvironment where cells secrete and regulate various substances. The mucosal epithelium contains specialized cells, including:

Parietal cells: Secrete hydrochloric acid and intrinsic factor, essential for vitamin B12 absorption.

Chief cells: Produce pepsinogen, the precursor to pepsin.

Mucous neck cells: Generate mucus and bicarbonate, forming the primary defense against the acidic gastric content.

G cells: Release gastrin, a hormone that stimulates acid secretion.

Gastric Mucosal Defense and Repair
The stomach has an incredible ability to protect itself from its own digestive juices. This is achieved through:

- Tight junctions between epithelial cells, preventing leaks.

- Rapid cell turnover, with new cells replacing damaged ones.
- Blood flow, which removes acid and provides nutrients for repair.
- Prostaglandins, which promote mucus and bicarbonate production and ensure adequate blood flow.

Interactions with the Nervous System

The enteric nervous system, often called the "second brain," governs the stomach's motility and secretory functions. It works in concert with the central nervous system, responding to stress and emotions, which can influence gastric function.

Hormonal Regulation

The stomach's activity is tightly regulated by hormones like gastrin, ghrelin, and somatostatin, which control hunger, satiety, and acid secretion. These hormones interact with other organs, such as the pancreas and the small intestine, to coordinate digestion.

Immune Function in the Gastric Mucosa
The stomach also plays a role in immunity. The gastric mucosa contains immune cells that can detect and respond to pathogens, providing a first line of defense against ingested microbes.

This chapter has explored the complex environment of the stomach and its interactions with other organs. Understanding this intricate system is crucial for grasping the pathogenesis of gastric ulcers and the broader implications for digestive health. The subsequent chapters will build upon this knowledge, focusing on the pathological changes that lead to ulcer formation and the strategies employed to combat this ailment.

In summary, the gastric environment is a complex system that balances aggressive digestive processes with protective mechanisms. Its relationship with other internal organs is crucial for the proper digestion and absorption of nutrients. Understanding this intricate balance is key to comprehending the pathogenesis of gastric ulcers and their treatment.

Chapter 3: Pathophysiology of Gastric Ulcers

Gastric ulcers, a subtype of peptic ulcers, are lesions that form in the stomach lining. Understanding their pathophysiology is crucial for effective treatment and prevention. This chapter delves into the causes, risk factors, and the intricate role of Helicobacter pylori in the development of these ulcers, as well as the impact of stress and lifestyle choices.

Causes and Risk Factors

Genetic Predisposition
Research indicates that individuals with a family history of gastric ulcers are at a higher risk. For example, a study might find that a particular

Gene variant, associated with increased gastric acid production, is more prevalent in patients with gastric ulcers.

Environmental Factors

Lifestyle choices significantly impact ulcer risk. For instance, a diet high in spicy foods can exacerbate gastric irritation, while alcohol and smoking can impair the stomach lining's ability to repair itself.

Medications

The widespread use of **NSAIDs** for pain relief has been linked to increased ulcer risk. A case study might describe a patient who developed an ulcer after prolonged **NSAID** use for arthritis.

Physiological Stress

The stress-ulcer syndrome is well-documented in critically ill patients. For example, a patient may develop stress-related ulcers following major surgery due to the body's heightened physiological response.

The Role of H. pylori

Discovery and Characteristics of H. pylori
The bacterium was discovered by Barry Marshall and Robin Warren, who demonstrated its role in gastritis and ulcer disease. They famously self-experimented to prove causation.

Mechanisms of Mucosal Damage

H. pylori produces urease, which converts urea to ammonia, neutralizing stomach acid and allowing the bacteria to thrive. The presence of CagA increases the risk of severe gastric inflammation and ulceration.

Immune Response to H. pylori

The immune system's attempt to eradicate *H. pylori* can lead to chronic gastritis. For instance, a biopsy might show lymphocytes and plasma cells infiltrating the gastric mucosa, indicative of an immune response.

Treatment Strategies

The standard treatment, known as triple therapy, includes two antibiotics and a proton pump inhibitor. Success stories include patients who have achieved complete ulcer healing following this regimen.

Stress and Lifestyle Contributions

Psychological Stress

The case of a high-stress executive developing an ulcer during a particularly stressful quarter illustrates the impact of psychological stress on gastric health.

Lifestyle Factors

Conversely, a study might show that individuals who engage in regular moderate exercise have a lower incidence of gastric ulcers, suggesting a protective effect.

Dietary Influences

Antioxidant-rich foods like berries and green tea have been shown to reduce oxidative stress in the gastric mucosa, potentially lowering ulcer risk.

Complications of gastric ulcers can be serious and sometimes life-threatening. Some of the main complications include:

complication of gastric ulcer

Internal Bleeding: This can occur when an ulcer develops at the site of a blood vessel, leading to anemia or severe blood loss that may require hospitalization and blood transfusion.

Perforation: A rarer but very serious complication where the stomach lining splits open, allowing bacteria to infect the abdominal cavity (peritonitis), which can lead to sepsis and multiple organ failure if untreated.

Gastric Outlet Obstruction: An inflamed or scarred ulcer can block food from moving through the digestive system, causing vomiting, bloating, and weight loss.

It's important to seek medical attention if experiencing symptoms like severe stomach pain, vomiting blood, or black, tarry stools, as these may indicate complications from a gastric ulcer.

Chapter 4: Symptoms and Diagnosis

The Importance of Early Diagnosis
Early diagnosis of gastric ulcers is crucial as it can prevent complications and lead to more effective treatment. Recognizing the early signs and symptoms can significantly improve patient outcome

Recognizing the Signs

The common symptoms of gastric ulcers include:
- Persistent stomach pain
- Bloating
- Heartburn
- Nausea

Patients may also experience vomiting, which can sometimes contain blood, indicating a more severe condition.

Appropriate Measures in the Early Stage

Upon noticing symptoms, individuals should:

- Consult a healthcare provider promptly.
- Avoid irritants such as NSAIDs, alcohol, and smoking.
- Adopt dietary changes to avoid foods that exacerbate symptoms.

Diagnostic Tools and Techniques

Modern diagnostic methods include:

- Endoscopy A procedure where a camera is inserted into the stomach to visualize ulcers.
- **Barium Swallow X-ray**: A radiographic examination that helps visualize the stomach lining.

- **H. pylori Testing**: Blood, breath, and
  stool tests to detect the presence of **H.
  pylori** bacteria.

**Traditional methods, though less common
now, included:**
- **Dietary Analysis:** Observing symptom
  patterns in response to dietary changes.
- **Physical Examination:** Palpation and
  auscultation to detect abnormalities.

Differential Diagnosis

Differential diagnosis involves distinguishing
gastric ulcers from other conditions with similar
symptoms, such as:
- Gastric cancer
- Gastroesophageal reflux disease (GERD)
- Gastritis

For example, while both gastric cancer and ulcers can cause stomach pain, cancer may also present with weight loss and fatigue.
A case study might describe a patient who presented with stomach pain and bloating, initially suspected to have GERD, but was later diagnosed with a gastric ulcer through endoscopy.

Illustrations could include endoscopic images of a gastric ulcer, charts comparing symptoms of differential diagnoses, and diagrams of diagnostic procedures.

This chapter provides a comprehensive overview of the symptoms and diagnostic approaches for gastric ulcers, emphasizing the importance of early detection and accurate diagnosis.

Role of diet in managing gastric ulcer

Diet plays a significant role in managing gastric ulcers, both in alleviating symptoms and in aiding the healing process.

Here's how diet can help:

Alleviating Symptoms: Certain foods can help soothe the stomach lining and reduce acid production, which may alleviate the pain and discomfort associated with gastric ulcers[1].

Fighting H. pylori: Some foods contain compounds that may help fight against *Helicobacter pylori* (H. pylori), the bacteria often responsible for causing ulcers. Foods rich in antioxidants, such as blueberries, cherries, and bell peppers, can support the immune system in combating this infection[1].

Promoting Healing: A diet rich in fiber and certain vitamins can promote healing of the stomach lining. Foods high in vitamin A and fiber, for example, has been shown to reduce the risk of peptic ulcers.

Probiotics: Fermented foods containing probiotics, like yogurt and kefir, can help maintain a healthy balance of gut bacteria and may be beneficial in managing H. pylori infections.

It's important to note that while diet can support ulcer treatment, it should be used in conjunction with appropriate medical therapies prescribed by healthcare professionals. Avoiding irritants like spicy foods, alcohol, and smoking is also crucial in managing gastric ulcers effectively.

Chapter 5: Medical Treatment Strategies

Pharmacological Interventions

Pharmacological interventions for gastric ulcers aim to promote healing by reducing gastric acid secretion and enhancing mucosal defense mechanisms. The main classes of drugs used include:

Proton Pump Inhibitors (PPIs): These are the most potent inhibitors of acid secretion. They work by irreversibly blocking the H+/K+ ATPase enzyme system of the gastric parietal cells.

H2 Receptor Antagonists: These reduce acid secretion by blocking histamine action on H2 receptors of gastric parietal cells.

Antacids: These neutralize existing stomach acid and provide rapid but short-term relief of symptoms.

Mucosal Protective Agents: Drugs like sucralfate and bismuth subsalicylate form a protective barrier over the ulcer site, protecting it from acid and pepsin.

Antibiotic Therapies

Antibiotic therapies are crucial when Helicobacter pylori infection is present, as this bacterium is a common cause of gastric ulcers. A combination of antibiotics, usually two or three, is used to ensure the eradication of the bacterium. Common antibiotics include:

- Amoxicillin
- Clarithromycin
- Metronidazole
- Tetracycline

These are often prescribed alongside a PPI to increase treatment efficacy.

Acid Suppression and its Mechanisms
Acid suppression therapy is central to the treatment of gastric ulcers.

The mechanisms include:
Decreasing Gastric Acid Secretion: PPIs and H2 receptor antagonists lower acid production.

Neutralizing Gastric Acid: Antacids neutralize the acid in the stomach, providing symptomatic relief.

 Enhancing Mucosal Defenses: Drugs that increase the production of mucus and bicarbonate help strengthen the stomach lining against acid attack.

The goal of these strategies is to create an environment conducive to healing the ulcer and preventing recurrence.

Integrative and Adjunctive Therapies
Dietary Modifications: Although no specific diet can cure ulcers, avoiding foods that irritate the stomach lining may help symptoms.
Stress Management: Techniques like meditation, yoga, and cognitive-behavioral therapy can help manage stress, which may exacerbate ulcer symptoms.

Monitoring and Follow-Up
Endoscopic Evaluation: Regular endoscopy can monitor healing and detect potential complications like bleeding or perforation.
Treatment Adjustment: Based on response and side effects, treatment regimens may need adjustments over time.

Patient Education
Medication Adherence: Patients should be educated on the importance of completing the full course of medications, even if symptoms improve.

Lifestyle Changes: Smoking cessation and limiting alcohol can significantly impact the healing process and prevent recurrence.

The medications used for treating gastric ulcers can have a range of side effects. Here are some common ones associated with each type of medication:

Proton Pump Inhibitors (PPIs)
- Headache
- Diarrhea or constipation
- Nausea
- Abdominal pain
- Fatigue

H2 Receptor Antagonists
- Headaches
- Dizziness
- Diarrhea
- Constipation
- Muscle pain

Antacids

- Diarrhea (magnesium-containing antacids)
- Constipation (aluminum-containing antacids)
- Calcium carbonate can cause kidney stones if taken in large doses

Antibiotics

- Nausea and vomiting
- Diarrhea
- A metallic taste in the mouth
- Discoloration of the tongue

Mucosal Protective Agents

- Constipation (for drugs like sucralfate)
- Changes in bowel movements

Cytoprotective Agents

- Gas
- Dry mouth
- Headache

It's important to note that while these are common side effects, not everyone will experience them, and some individuals may experience side effects not listed here. If side effects are severe or persistent, it's crucial to consult a healthcare provider. Always use medications as prescribed and report any adverse reactions to your doctor.

Chapter 6: Surgical Interventions

Surgical intervention for gastric ulcers is typically considered when medical therapy is insufficient or complications arise. Surgery can address the ulcer directly, control stomach acid production, and prevent further complications.

Indications for Surgery

Surgery may be indicated in the following scenarios:

- **Non-healing Ulcers**: Persistent ulcers that do not heal with medical treatment.
- **Bleeding**: When an ulcer leads to significant or recurrent bleeding.

- **Perforation**: If the ulcer creates a hole in the stomach wall.
- **Obstruction:** When an ulcer blocks the passage of food through the digestive tract.
- **Cancer Suspicions**: If there's a possibility the ulcer is malignant.
- **Intractable Pain**: Severe ulcer pain not relieved by medication.
- **Suspicion of Malignancy**: If there's a concern that the ulcer could be cancerous, surgery may be necessary for diagnosis and treatment.

Patients should look out for signs like sharp, persistent stomach pain, blood in vomit or stool, unexplained weight loss, and severe nausea or vomiting as indicators for potential surgery.

Types of Surgical Procedures

Surgical Techniques and Advances

Surgical interventions have evolved to minimize invasiveness and improve recovery times. Techniques include:

- **Laparoscopic Surgery**: Small incisions and specialized instruments are used to perform the surgery, leading to faster recovery and less pain.
- **Endoscopic Procedures**: For certain complications like bleeding, endoscopic techniques can be used to treat ulcers without external incisions.

- **Billroth I (Gastroduodenostomy)**: The lower part of the stomach is removed, and the remainder is connected to the duodenum.

- **Billroth II (Gastrojejunostomy)**: The lower part of the stomach is removed, and the remainder is connected to the jejunum.

- **Vagotomy**:Cutting the vagus nerve to reduce acid secretion.
- **Antrectomy**: Removing the lower part of the stomach that produces gastrin.
- **Pyloroplasty**: Enlarging the opening of the pylorus to improve stomach emptying.
- **Gastrectomy**: Partial or total removal of the stomach.
- **Graham Patch**:Covering a perforation with omental tissue.

Each procedure has specific indications and is chosen based on the patient's condition and the ulcer's characteristics.

Postoperative Care

Postoperative care includes:
Pain Management: Using medications to control pain.
Diet: Starting with liquid foods and gradually reintroducing solids.

Activity: Encouraging movement to prevent complications like deep vein thrombosis.

Monitoring: Regular check-ups to ensure proper healing and to detect any complications early.

Nutritional Support: Some patients may require nutritional support via a feeding tube or intravenously until they can eat normally.

Rehabilitation: Physical therapy may be needed to regain strength and mobility.
Complications of Gastric Ulcer Surgery

Complications can include:

Infection:At the surgical site or within the abdomen.

 Bleeding:Which may require transfusion or additional surgery.

Anastomotic Leak:Leakage at the surgical connection between stomach and intestine.

Nutritional Deficiencies:Due to altered digestion and absorption.

Dumping Syndrome: Rapid gastric emptying causing nausea, weakness, and sweating.

Post-Vagotomy Diarrhea: Increased frequency and liquidity of bowel movements.

Recurrence of Ulcers: Despite successful surgery, ulcers can recur and may require further treatment.

Surgical interventions are a critical component in managing complex cases of gastric ulcers. They offer a solution to life-threatening complications and provide a path to recovery when other treatments fail.

Before undergoing gastric ulcer surgery, it's important to have a clear understanding of the procedure, its risks, and the expected outcomes.

Here are some common questions you might consider asking your surgeon:

1. What are the indications for this surgery in my case?
2. What are the different surgical options available, and which do you recommend?
3. How is the surgery performed, and what techniques will be used?
4. What are the potential risks and complications of the surgery?
5. How long is the recovery period, and what kind of postoperative care will I need?
6. What lifestyle changes or dietary restrictions will I need to follow after the surgery?
7. Are there any alternatives to surgery that I should consider?

8. How will this surgery affect my overall health and quality of life?
9. What is your experience with this type of surgery, and what are the success rates?
10. Can I speak with patients who have undergone the same surgery?

These questions can help you make an informed decision and prepare for the surgery and its aftermath. Remember, it's crucial to communicate openly with your healthcare team and ensure all your concerns are addressed before proceeding with any surgical intervention.

Chapter 7: Nutritional Considerations and Lifestyle Modifications

The Association Between Diet and Gastric Ulcers: Misconceptions and Facts

Gastric ulcers, once thought to be primarily caused by stress and spicy foods, are now better understood. The role of diet in the development and management of gastric ulcers is nuanced, and several misconceptions persist. Here's what current research tells us:

Misconceptions:
Spicy Foods Cause Ulcers: While spicy foods can irritate the stomach lining, they are not a cause of gastric ulcers.

Ulcers Are Caused by Stress Alone: Stress may exacerbate symptoms, but it is not the sole cause of ulcers. The primary cause is the bacterium Helicobacter pylori, along with the use of certain medications.

Milk Can Heal Ulcers: Drinking milk may provide temporary relief by coating the stomach lining, but it does not heal ulcers and can actually increase stomach acid production.

Facts:

H. pylori Infection: A significant cause of ulcers, this bacterium can be influenced by dietary factors. Foods rich in antioxidants may help the body fight the infection.

Dietary Impact:There is no specific ulcer diet, but certain foods may help manage symptoms and support healing. These include foods rich in flavonoids, probiotics, and a balanced intake of fiber.

Foods to Avoid: It's recommended to avoid foods that irritate the stomach or increase acid production, such as alcohol, caffeine, and fatty foods.

In summary, while diet alone is not responsible for causing or curing gastric ulcers, it plays a supportive role in managing symptoms and promoting healing. Understanding the balance between myths and evidence-based facts can help individuals make informed dietary choices in conjunction with medical treatment for gastric ulcers.

Diet and Gastric Health

A balanced diet plays a crucial role in maintaining gastric health and aiding the healing process of gastric ulcers.

The focus should be on:

High Fiber Foods: Whole grains, fruits, vegetables, and beans can help reduce the chance of developing gastritis and promote gut health.

Low Fat Foods: Fish, lean meats, and vegetables are easier to digest and less likely to irritate the stomach lining.

Foods with Low Acidity: Including more vegetables and beans in the diet can prevent irritation of the gastric mucosa.

Probiotics: Foods like yogurt, kefir, and sauerkraut can help maintain a healthy balance of gut bacteria, which is essential for digestive health.

Foods to Avoid and Why
Certain foods can exacerbate gastric ulcer symptoms or contribute to their development:

Spicy Foods: Can irritate the stomach lining and worsen pain and inflammation.

Acidic Foods: Tomatoes and citrus fruits can increase stomach acidity and irritate existing ulcers.

Caffeinated Beverages: Coffee (even decaf) and certain sodas can stimulate acid production.

Alcohol: Can damage the mucosal lining and increase the risk of bleeding.

Fatty Foods: High-fat meals can slow down digestion and increase the risk of acid reflux.

Stress Management Techniques
Stress can significantly impact gastric health, exacerbating symptoms and delaying healing. Effective stress management techniques include:

Yoga and Meditation: These practices can improve digestion and reduce stress-related inflammation in the gut.

Regular Exercise: Physical activity can help manage stress and promote overall digestive health.

Mindful Eating: Taking the time to eat slowly and without distractions can improve digestion and reduce stress levels.

Adequate Sleep: Ensuring sufficient rest can help manage stress and improve the body's healing processes.

Incorporating these dietary and lifestyle changes can lead to better management of gastric ulcers and overall digestive health. It's important to consult with healthcare professionals before making significant changes to diet or lifestyle, especially when managing a condition like gastric ulcers.

Exercise can play a beneficial role in managing gastric ulcers through several mechanisms:

1. Enhancing Immune Function: Regular moderate exercise may improve the body's immune response, which could help neutralize the effects of H. pylori, a common bacterium associated with gastric ulcers.

2. Reducing Acid Secretion: Physical activity might influence the stomach's acid production, potentially reducing excess acid secretion that can aggravate ulcers.

3. Stress Reduction: Exercise is known to help reduce stress, which can be a contributing factor to the development and exacerbation of gastric ulcers. By managing stress, the overall impact on gastric health can be positive.

4. Promoting Healthy Lifestyle Choices: Engaging in regular physical activity can encourage other healthy behaviors, such as a balanced diet and avoiding harmful habits like smoking and excessive alcohol consumption, which are risk factors for ulcer development.

It's important to note that while moderate exercise can be beneficial, intense physical activity might have adverse effects, such as suppressing immune function and reducing mucosal blood flow, which could potentially worsen ulcer conditions. Therefore, it's recommended to maintain a balance and opt for moderate, regular exercise.

Always consult with a healthcare provider before starting any new exercise regimen, especially if you have a medical condition like gastric ulcers. They can provide guidance on the most appropriate type and amount of exercise for your specific situation.

Chapter 8: Alternative Therapies for Gastric Ulcer

Gastric ulcers, a type of peptic ulcer, are lesions in the stomach lining. The conventional treatment involves medications that reduce stomach acid and antibiotics to treat H. pylori infections. However, alternative therapies can complement traditional treatments, offering holistic relief and healing. This chapter delves into three such therapies: herbal remedies, acupuncture and acupressure, and mind-body approaches.

Herbal Remedies and Preparation

Herbal remedies have been used for centuries to treat a variety of ailments, including gastric ulcers. They offer a natural way to support the body's healing processes.

Cabbage Juice: Rich in vitamin C and glutamine, cabbage juice promotes healing of the stomach lining. To prepare, blend fresh cabbage with water and drink the juice immediately.

Licorice Root: DGL (licorice) can soothe the stomach lining and aid in

Honey: Known for its antibacterial properties, honey can inhibit the growth of H. pylori. Incorporate it into your diet or take a spoonful on an empty stomach.

Aloe Vera: Aloe vera juice may help reduce inflammation in the stomach. Drink a small amount of aloe vera juice daily, ensuring it's free from aloin, which can be a laxative.

Acupuncture and Acupressure

Acupuncture and acupressure are components of Traditional Chinese Medicine (TCM) and can be effective in managing gastric ulcer symptoms.

Acupuncture: Involves inserting thin needles at specific points to balance the body's energy flow, or Qi. It may reduce ulcer pain and promote healing.

Acupressure: A non-invasive form of acupuncture, acupressure involves applying pressure to certain points on the body. It can be self-administered to relieve symptoms.

Mind-Body Approaches

Mind-body approaches focus on the connection between mental and physical health, emphasizing stress reduction and emotional well-being as a pathway to physical healing.

Meditation: Reduces stress, which is a known exacerbator of gastric ulcers. Practice mindfulness or guided meditation daily.

Yoga: Combines physical postures, breathing exercises, and meditation to promote relaxation and stress relief.

Biofeedback: Uses electronic monitoring to train individuals to control bodily processes that are normally involuntary, like heart rate, which can improve stress management.

These alternative therapies can be integrated into a comprehensive treatment plan for gastric ulcers. Always consult with a healthcare provider before starting any new treatment to ensure it's appropriate for your specific condition.

Conventional treatments for gastric ulcers typically involve a combination of medications aimed at reducing stomach acid and eradicating

any underlying infection, particularly H. pylori.

Here are some of the standard treatments:

- **Antibiotics**: If an H. pylori infection is present, a course of antibiotics is prescribed to eliminate the bacteria. Common antibiotics include amoxicillin, clarithromycin, metronidazole, tinidazole, tetracycline, and levofloxacin.

- **Proton Pump Inhibitors (PPIs)**: These medications reduce acid production in the stomach, which helps heal the ulcer and provide relief from symptoms. Examples are omeprazole, lansoprazole, rabeprazole, esomeprazole, and pantoprazole.

- **H2 Blockers**: Similar to PPIs, H2
  blockers also reduce stomach acid and are
  used in the treatment of gastric ulcers.

- **Bismuth Subsalicylate**: This medication
  can protect the stomach lining and may be
  used alongside other treatments.

Antacids: These can provide quick relief by
neutralizing stomach acid.
It's important to follow the treatment plan
prescribed by a healthcare provider, as the
effectiveness of these treatments can depend on
factors such as the cause of the ulcer and the
individual's overall health[2]. Additionally,
lifestyle changes, such as quitting smoking and
avoiding NSAIDs, can help prevent ulcers from
worsening or recurring.

Chapter 9: Complications and Management of Gastric Ulcers

Gastric ulcers can lead to serious complications if not managed properly. This chapter outlines the major complications associated with gastric ulcers and their management strategies.

Bleeding Ulcers

Bleeding is one of the most common complications of gastric ulcers. It can range from minor bleeding, which may go unnoticed, to severe hemorrhage, presenting as melena (black, tarry stools) or hematemesis (vomiting blood).

Management

Endoscopic Therapy: For active bleeding, endoscopic interventions such as thermal coagulation, injection of epinephrine, or application of hemostatic clips can be used.

Medication: Proton pump inhibitors (PPIs) are administered to reduce acid production and facilitate healing.

Surgery: In cases where bleeding cannot be controlled endoscopically, surgical intervention may be necessary.

Perforation and Penetration
Perforation occurs when an ulcer creates a hole in the stomach wall, leading to peritonitis, an inflammation of the peritoneum. Penetration happens when an ulcer extends into adjacent organs such as the pancreas.

Management
Immediate Surgery: Surgical repair is required to close the perforation and clean the abdominal cavity.

Antibiotics: Broad-spectrum antibiotics are administered to prevent or treat infection resulting from leakage of gastric contents into the peritoneal cavity.

Gastric Cancer Risks

Long-standing gastric ulcers can increase the risk of developing gastric cancer, especially if associated with chronic H. pylori infection.

Management

Regular Surveillance: Patients with gastric ulcers should undergo periodic endoscopic surveillance with biopsies to detect any malignant changes early.

Eradication of H. pylori: Treatment of H. pylori infection has been shown to reduce the risk of gastric cancer.

Certainly! Let's expand on the management of gastric ulcer complications with additional details.

Stricture Formation

A stricture is a narrowing of the stomach outlet that can occur after chronic inflammation and scarring from an ulcer.

Management

Endoscopic Dilation: This procedure involves stretching the narrowed area with a balloon or dilator to improve gastric emptying.

Surgery: In severe cases, surgical intervention may be required to remove the structure and reconstruct the affected area.

Gastrointestinal Obstruction

Gastrointestinal obstruction can occur when an ulcer leads to swelling or scarring that blocks the passage of food through the digestive tract.

Management
Nasogastric Tube: Insertion of a tube can relieve pressure and remove stomach contents.

Endoscopic Stent Placement: A stent may be placed to keep the passageway open.

surgery: Surgical procedures may be necessary to remove the obstruction.

Impact on Quality of Life
Gastric ulcers can significantly affect a patient's quality of life, causing pain, discomfort, and anxiety about eating.

Management
Dietary Changes: Eating smaller, more frequent meals and avoiding foods that irritate the stomach can help manage symptoms.

Pain Management: Use of medications and techniques to control pain and improve comfort.

Psychological Support: Counseling and support groups can help patients cope with the emotional impact of their condition.

Preventive Measures
Regular Monitoring: Regular check-ups and monitoring can help catch complications early.

Lifestyle Modifications: Avoiding smoking, reducing alcohol intake, and managing stress can help prevent ulcer formation and complications.

The management of gastric ulcer complications is multifaceted, involving both medical and lifestyle interventions. It's essential for patients to work closely with their healthcare providers to develop a personalized plan that addresses their specific needs and improves their overall well-being.

Also the management of complications associated with gastric ulcers requires a multidisciplinary approach involving gastroenterologists, surgeons, and oncologists. Prompt recognition and treatment of these complications are crucial for improving patient outcomes. Regular follow-ups and lifestyle modifications can also play a significant role in the management and prevention of these serious complications.

Chapter 10: The Future of Gastric Ulcer Management

The management of gastric ulcers is an evolving field, with ongoing research and clinical trials paving the way for innovative treatments and preventative strategies. This chapter explores the promising horizons in gastric ulcer management.

Ongoing Research and Clinical Trials
Research into gastric ulcers is continuously uncovering new insights into their pathophysiology, leading to more effective treatments. Clinical trials are investigating various aspects, including:

Helicobacter pylori Eradication: New regimens and combinations of antibiotics are being tested to overcome resistance and improve eradication rates.

Genetic Factors: Studies are exploring the genetic predisposition to ulcer formation and how this knowledge can lead to personalized medicine approaches.

Probiotics: The role of probiotics in managing gastric ulcers is under investigation, focusing on their potential to enhance mucosal defense and inhibit H. pylori.

Innovations in Treatment

Advancements in treatment options are being developed to provide better outcomes for patients with gastric ulcers:

Vonoprazan: A new class of potent acid inhibitors, known as potassium-competitive acid blockers (P-CABs), is showing promise in treating acid-related disorders, including gastric ulcers[1].

Stem Cell Therapy: Preliminary research into stem cell therapy offers hope for regenerating damaged gastric mucosa and providing a cure for chronic ulcers.

Preventative Strategies

Preventative strategies for gastric ulcers are crucial in reducing the incidence and severity of the disease. Here are some extended strategies that are currently being explored:

Prevention is key in managing gastric ulcers. Emerging strategies include:

Diet and Lifestyle: Emphasizing a diet rich in fruits, vegetables, and whole grains while avoiding NSAIDs and managing stress effectively.

Screening and Early Detection: Identifying at-risk individuals through non-invasive testing and initiating early treatment to prevent ulcer formation.

 Education: Increasing awareness about the risk factors and symptoms of gastric ulcers to promote early intervention.

Lifestyle Modifications: Beyond diet and stress management, researchers are looking into the impact of sleep patterns and physical activity on ulcer prevention.

Microbiome Analysis: Understanding the role of the gut microbiome in gastric health could lead to probiotic treatments that prevent ulcer formation.

Genetic Screening: Identifying individuals with a genetic predisposition to ulcers may allow for early intervention and personalized preventative measures.

Vaccination: There is ongoing research into the development of a vaccine against H. pylori, which could provide a long-term solution to preventing gastric ulcers.

Public Health Initiatives: Education campaigns to raise awareness about the causes and prevention of gastric ulcers, especially in regions with high H. pylori prevalence.

The future of gastric ulcer management looks promising, with research and innovation leading to more effective and personalized treatment options. Preventative measures will play a crucial role in reducing the incidence and complications associated with this condition. As we look ahead, a multidisciplinary approach involving gastroenterologists, researchers, and patients will be essential in realizing these advancements.

Conclusion:

Embracing the Journey to Healing

As we close the pages of this book, **"The Art and Science of Gastric Ulcer: Acidic Alchemy,"** we reflect on the journey we've embarked upon—a journey that intertwines the delicate threads of medical science with the rich tapestry of holistic healing. Gastric ulcers, a testament to the complexities of the human body, challenge us to look beyond the symptoms and to understand the intricate dance between health and disease.

Through the chapters, we've explored the depths of conventional treatments and the promise of alternative therapies, each offering a beacon of hope for those navigating the turbulent waters of gastric discomfort. We've delved into the complications and management strategies, acknowledging the shadows cast by potential risks while illuminating the paths to recovery.

The future of gastric ulcer management shines bright with the light of ongoing research, clinical trials, and innovations in treatment. Preventative strategies stand as sentinels, guarding against the recurrence of this ailment and empowering individuals with the knowledge and tools to maintain their well-being.

In this odyssey of healing, we are reminded that the management of gastric ulcers is not a solitary pursuit but a collective endeavor. It is a symphony composed by the dedicated hands of healthcare professionals, the inquisitive minds of researchers, and the resilient spirits of patients.

Let this book serve as a compass for those seeking solace from gastric pain, a map leading to the treasure trove of health. May the art and science of managing gastric ulcers continue to evolve, as we, too, grow in our understanding and capability to nurture the body's innate ability to heal.

In the grand alchemy of life, where acid and enzyme mix, let us find the elixir of health, the ultimate fix. For in the balance of body and mind lies the greatest discovery: that the truest form of healing comes from harmony within.

And so, we step forward, with knowledge as our guide, embracing the art and science of gastric ulcers, side by side.

If you got value kindly leave a positive review
and Also check out my others books here:
https://www.amazon.com/author/elvygraves

www.ingramcontent.com/pod-product-compliance
Lightning Source LLC
Chambersburg PA
CBHW050828250726
48653CB00006B/2480